I0434377

POCDOC

POCDOC

POCKET DOCTOR

DR. GREGORY KIMMERLE

iUniverse, Inc.
Bloomington

PocDoc
Pocket Doctor

Copyright © 2011 by Dr. Gregory Kimmerle.

All rights reserved. No part of this book may be used or reproduced by any means, graphic, electronic, or mechanical, including photocopying, recording, taping or by any information storage retrieval system without the written permission of the publisher except in the case of brief quotations embodied in critical articles and reviews.

iUniverse books may be ordered through booksellers or by contacting:

iUniverse
1663 Liberty Drive
Bloomington, IN 47403
www.iuniverse.com
1-800-Authors (1-800-288-4677)

Because of the dynamic nature of the Internet, any web addresses or links contained in this book may have changed since publication and may no longer be valid. The views expressed in this work are solely those of the author and do not necessarily reflect the views of the publisher, and the publisher hereby disclaims any responsibility for them.

Any people depicted in stock imagery provided by Thinkstock are models, and such images are being used for illustrative purposes only.

Certain stock imagery © Thinkstock.

ISBN: 978-1-4620-4501-3 (sc)
ISBN: 978-1-4620-4282-1 (ebk)

Library of Congress Control Number: 2011914237

Printed in the United States of America

iUniverse rev. date: 08/10/2011

CONTENTS

Disclaimer

This book is for adults only. Though I am a board-certified physician and I am not your doctor, I believe I can be of great assistance in lengthening your life. By opening this book, you agree—unconditionally—to consult your doctor on all of the following topics before any changes are made. If you don't have a personal doctor that you see regularly, get one now. Your personal physician and you will be the team ultimately responsible for your healthcare decisions. There are no excuses for not taking care of yourself. The material inside is easy to understand; but as we all know, changing ourselves is the difficult part.

Prologue

Why are you reading this book? Life is somewhat of a gamble; there are some things we can change or predict—and some things we cannot. We can predict the most common causes of death. By reading and applying what you read in this book, I believe that you will decrease your chances of dying from the most likely killers in the USA. This means you get to see more grandchildren, family, graduations, weddings, and life. Your doctors also know these topics, but the reality of medicine in this country is that it is hectic and sometimes disconnected. They may or may not have told you—or they may have tried, but had to address another topic or three during your office visit.

A recurring theme that you may notice in this book is diet, exercise, healthy weight maintenance, and healthy lifestyle. I have seen this formula applied in various patients—and even in family members—over the years, resulting in great success. Following the above lifestyle, my own grandmother lived independently in her own two-story home well into her upper nineties.

Her daily routine included yoga; healthy snacks, including almonds and green tea; and Bible studies for mental exercise. This type of background colored my perception of medicine to one that should be more proactive and thus strive to prevent disease. This book attempts to communicate this proactive belief with the hope that you will learn—and use—easy-to-remember guidelines based on facts. There will be references that you may look up to verify statements. By knowing your blood pressure and cholesterol goals—and the times at which cancer screening is recommended—you will at least decrease your risk of the three most common killers: **heart attack, cancer, and stroke.**[1]

As you may have gathered from the title, this book was intentionally made small and portable. I hope that you take advantage of this portability and bring this book as a reference to some of your medical appointments.

Your Heart

Let's simplify this complex organ. The heart is a muscle that pumps your blood. Like many pumps or engines, it has fuel lines, or arteries. If the fuel lines are blocked, the engine malfunctions or stops and there is no blood flow or life. It is important to keep the fuel lines wide open. Three things do this in a major way: **controlling blood pressure, controlling cholesterol, and not smoking**.

Nobody's Cancer

Unfortunately, anyone can get cancer. However, certain healthy behaviors and periodic tests can decrease the risk of cancer-related death—sometimes by 33 percent.[1] (K=1,000 people/year)

The Top Four Causes of Death by Cancer[3]

Men	Women
1. Lung (86.22K)	1. Lung (71.08K)
2. Prostate (32.05K)	2. Breast (39.84K)
3. Colorectal (26.58K)	3. Colorectal (24.79K)
4. Pancreatic (18.77K)	4. Pancreatic (18.03K)

Follow these guidelines[4] and obviously do not smoke:

- Men should have a prostate examination and a blood test called a PSA at age forty if you are of African descent or otherwise at higher risk (for example, a family history of prostate cancer). You may have it checked at fifty years of age if you have no risk factors or symptoms of altered urinary function, and then annually thereafter. This test is best discussed with your doctor as it may not be indicated in some men, and it is a somewhat nonspecific test.

- Women should start annual mammograms at age forty, or earlier if there are other risk factors or family history. Also, have your doctor show you how and when to self-examine.

- Have your colon checked at age fifty—or earlier if you have risk factors, family history, or symptoms. Discuss your family history and risk factors with your doctor.

- Be as lean as possible within your healthy/normal range of body weight.

- Be physically active as part of everyday life.

- Limit consumption of energy-dense foods and candy—and avoid sugary drinks.

- Eat mostly foods of plant origin.

- Limit intake of red meat and avoid eating processed meat.
- Limit alcoholic drinks.
- Limit consumption of salty processed foods. Avoid moldy cereals (grains) and legumes that can produce carcinogenic compounds that are not very common in the USA.
- Aim to meet nutritional needs through diet alone (rather than with supplements).
- Mothers should breastfeed.
- Cancer survivors should follow the recommendations for cancer prevention and screening.

The above may reduce your risk of cancer by one-third. If you stop tobacco use, it is possible that more than half of all cancers could be prevented.[2] Use sunblock and limit sun exposure between nine o'clock and three o'clock. This would decrease the risk of the most common cancer, which is skin cancer of the non-melanoma type (>1,000,000K). Since this type of cancer is not typically lethal, it was not listed above.

Your Brain

The third leading cause of death in the United States is stroke. To decrease your risk, control your blood pressure (below 140/90), keep your cholesterol at the level recommended by your physician, and control your blood sugar. Smoking should never be started—or it should be stopped as soon as possible.

Blood Pressure

As you may have guessed, controlling blood pressure is essential. Everyone should be less than 140/90; certain populations, such as diabetics, should be less than 130/80.

The first line of defense against high blood pressure should be a low-sodium (salt) diet, exercise as recommended by your MD, and weight loss if appropriate.[5]

If the above do not lead to adequate control within six months, medications should be prescribed by your doctor. Here are some of the preferred choices:

- Diuretics (like hydrochlorothiazide) are often a first choice. They decrease slight elevations in blood pressure, but can lower potassium levels, and possibly worsen gout. Blood tests are needed after starting the medicine. As always, discuss possible side effects with your doctor.

- Angiotensin-converting enzyme inhibitors (ACE-inhibitors, like lisinopril) are also excellent and preferred in diabetics, and those who have had strokes, heart attacks, or heart failure. They may cause a cough. Blood tests are needed after starting or increasing the medicine. ACE-inhibitors are to be avoided during pregnancy.

- Beta-blockers (like metoprolol) are great and preferred in patients after a heart attack. They can slow the heart rate, worsen asthma and emphysema (COPD), and cause—or worsen—depression and erectile dysfunction.

- Calcium channel-blockers (like amlodipine or diltiazem) are also good—and sometimes preferred—in African Americans. Some can slow the heart rate, cause constipation, or cause swelling.

Cholesterol

The description of cholesterol can be broken down into subtypes and numbers. Most people quote their total number, but the guidelines are based on the subtypes, especially the LDL (bad) and HDL (good) cholesterol numbers.

Your goal varies on your number of risk factors (in bullet points below). Some conditions or groups have a higher risk for heart attack:

- Males age 45 and over.
- Females age 55 and over.
- Smokers.
- Hypertension.
- First-degree male relatives with coronary heart disease before the age of fifty-five.

- First-degree female relative with coronary heart disease before the age of sixty-five.
- Having HDL levels less than forty.

Remember that LDL means keep it low, and HDL means keep it high. If you add up your risk factors, you are able to determine your goal LDL:

Risk factors	Goal LDL
0-1	<160
>/=2	<130

Diabetics, those who have had heart attacks, and coronary and peripheral artery disease patients should have a goal LDL of at least <100. Some diabetics and others with multiple risk factors have a goal LDL of <70. Goal cholesterol levels can also be determined with a cardiac risk calculator and the help of your physician.[7]

The treatment, of course, starts with a good diet—think vegetables, fruit, fiber, and fish for adults that are not pregnant. For many patients, medicines are also needed, and the statin class is the most effective. This includes atorvastatin (Lipitor®) and simvastatin (Zocor®). They reduce the liver's production of cholesterol and can be taken at night for greatest results. Discuss uncommon side effects and the need for periodic blood tests with your doctor. Attempt to keep the HDL >40 for men, and >50 for women through exercise, smoking cessation, or medication. Discuss with your doctor whether you should take a daily aspirin to help prevent stroke and heart attack.

Diabetes

Diabetes is rampant in the United States and abroad. Uncontrolled diabetes can damage the eyes, kidneys, and nerves—usually via small artery damage. Diet, weight loss, exercise, and medications can help control blood sugar. The medications—including, insulin, sulfonylureas, and biguanides—are best discussed with your doctor.

Consider following these recommendations:

- Keep your A1C <7.0 (for most diabetics), and check it at least biannually.
- Keep your LDL <100, or <70 for some people.
- Keep your blood pressure <130/80, preferably with the help of an ACE-inhibitor and check with your doctor at least biannually.
- Take an aspirin daily as directed by your doctor.

- Check your feet daily for sores, numbness, or signs of infection.
- Get your eyes checked annually by an eye-care specialist.
- Obtain a flu shot yearly.
- Receive a pneumonia vaccination as recommended by your doctor.
- Have your urine checked for protein at least yearly, looking for kidney disease.
- See a dietician or diabetic nurse.

The A1C is basically the average of your blood sugar over two or three months. It correlates to your home blood sugar as below.[8]

A1C	Average Blood Sugar
6%	126
7%	154
8%	183

Immunizations

Many immunizations and vaccinations are meant to prevent disease, infection, or cancer. Certain people should have them—your doctor will decide when to administer them.

- The first is the influenza vaccination or flu shot. People over fifty, diabetics, those with certain chronic lung conditions, and others should receive this every fall or winter.
- The pneumonia vaccination should be offered to those with diabetes, and other chronic diseases, people over sixty-five, and to those without a spleen.
- Hepatitis B vaccinations are given in three separate shots. It is recommended for all adolescents, people with liver disease, chronic kidney disease, and health care workers. This can decrease the risk of cirrhosis and liver cancer.

- Hepatitis A immunization is mostly for people with chronic liver disease, those that travel out of the "industrial" world, and certain subpopulations.
- The Tetanus/Diptheria/acellular Pertussis (TdaP) vaccine is for those who lack three previous doses, those with wounds (more than five years since their previous shot), and for a general booster every ten years. It is generally for people less than sixty-five and prevents whooping cough. For adults, this is a one-time dose after which the Td vaccination is offered.

Other shots help prevent chickenpox, meningitis, measles, mumps, rubella, shingles, and human papillomavirus, which can cause cancer in females.[9]

Diet

Your specific diet may need to be different if you're pregnant, have kidney stones, gout, or food allergies. Clear any new diet with your physician. It boils down to eating lots of vegetables and fruit, more fish, high fiber, and the right amounts of the right oils—and exercise. Colorful fruits and vegetables usually have a higher vitamin or mineral content. Vary the plant color by season for increased freshness and variety. Here are some guidelines:

EAT MORE	EAT LESS
colorful fresh clean veggies	potatoes, chips, french fries
fresh fruits	dried processed fruits
deep-water fish, skinless chicken	pork products
whole grains	processed white grains
nuts	candy
olive oil, canola oil	butter, margarine
herbs, spices, pepper	salt, sugar
water, skim milk, some fruit juices, green tea	coffee, soda, caffeine

Healthy Habits

- Don't smoke anything.
- Set aside time to exercise everyday for thirty minutes—or as your doctor directs.
- Drink a glass of filtered water and have some clean, raw vegetables or fruit before dinner so that you eat less of the "tastier" food.
- Brush your teeth at least twice per day and floss your teeth daily as this may improve your heart health.
- See your dentist as per their recommendations, which are often every six months.
- Have fun . . . at least once in a while.
- See your doctor as recommended.
- Men should periodically perform home testicular self-exams.

- Women should perform home breast self-exams, and go to the doctor for their scheduled pelvic exams and/or PAP smears.
- Limit alcohol consumption to one a day for women (greater amounts may increase your breast cancer risk). Men should limit consumption to a maximum of two a day.
- Avoid alcohol entirely if there is alcoholism in your family.
- Have your eyes checked regularly.
- Shop in the perimeter of the grocery store first. Buy your produce first, and then go to the interior where processed food is stored.
- Women over a certain age should consider supplemental calcium combined with vitamin D, and have bone strength checked as recommended by your doctor. Men may also consider a bone strength test if of a certain age, which is usually at seventy years.[10] Ask your doctor if any screening tests should be done in your particular case (such as an abdominal ultrasound in any male sixty-five to seventy-five that has a history of smoking, or is a current smoker). The goal is to catch things early if possible.

Conclusion

Please take the time to absorb at least some of the above material. If any of it resonates with you, you can use it to your advantage. If you have any questions or concerns, your doctor will be able to address them during your next office visit. Please take an active part in your own health and do some of your own research. Consult the Internet, the library, your friends, and your family, but take care of yourself.

The following pages are meant to be copied for your use. Please fill them out and consider carrying the page with the medication list with you at all times. Good luck, and see your personal physician so that as a team you may improve, or maintain your health. Together this team should decide if any changes should be made to your lifestyle, diet, or medications. This book is only a reference tool, and not a replacement for your doctor that knows your individual history, and who cares for your health.

✂ --- ✂

Personal Medical Records

My Medical Condition(s):

Date	BP	Date	BP	Date	BP	Date	BP	Date	BP

Date	LDL/HDL ... Cholesterol	A1C Diabetes	Urine Micro..	Creatinine Kidney	ALT Liver

Date	Mamm	Date	PAP	Date	PSA	Date	Colon

Date	"Shot"	Repeat in ...	Date	"Shot"	Repeat in ...

✂ --- ✂

Personal Medical Records

Medication	Dose	Frequency/When	Reason For taking

Allergies:

Date of Birth:	Durable Power of Attorney:	Advance Directives:

Physician	Specialty	Phone Number

✂ -- ✂

Personal Medical Records

Date	Surgery	Date	Surgery	Date	Surgery

My medical conditions:

Legend

A1C—Hemoglobin A1C, a blood test that reveals the average blood sugar control over approximately the last three months

BP—Blood pressure

Creat—Creatinine, a blood test that reflects kidney function

Colon—Colonoscopy, a procedure done via endoscopic visualization to screen for colon cancer

LDL/HDL—Low-density lipoprotein/high-density lipoprotein, two lab values that are used to monitor the level of cholesterol control

Liver—Shorthand for ALT/AST, which are two lab values that are checked periodically when one takes medications for lowering cholesterol

Mamm—Mammogram, a radiographic test used to detect breast cancer

Micro—Microalbumin, a urine test used to screen for protein in the urine that may lead to early detection of kidney dysfunction related to diabetes

PAP—The test result that shows the tissue obtained from females when screening for cervical cancer

PSA—Prostate specific antigen, a blood test done as a screening tool to detect prostate cancer

Shot—Vaccination

Bibliography

1. "CDC Health, United States, 2010: At a Glance Table," accessed April 25, 2011, http://www.cdc.gov/nchs/data/hus/hus10.pdf#glance

2. "American Cancer Society Guidelines on Nutrition and Physical Activity for Cancer Prevention," accessed April 25, 2011, http://caonline.amcancersoc.org/cgi/content/full/56/5/254?maxtoshow=&hits=10&RESULTFORMAT=&fulltext=prevention&searchid=1&FIRSTINDEX=0&resourcetype=HWCIT

3. "A Cancer Journal for Clinicians, Table 1 Estimated New Cancer Cases and Deaths by Sex, United States 2010," accessed April 25, 2011, http://caonline.amcancersoc.org/cgi/content-nw/full/60/5/277/TBL1

4. "American Institute for Cancer Research, Recommendations for cancer prevention, accessed April

25, 2011, http://www.aicr.org/site/PageServer?pagenam e=recommendations_home

5. "National High Blood Pressure Education Program, Table. 5," accessed April 26, 2011, http://www.nhlbi.nih. gov/guidelines/hypertension/express.pdf

6. "National Cholesterol Education Program, High Blood Cholesterol: What You Need to Know," accessed April 26, 2011, http://www.nhlbi.nih.gov/health/public/heart/ chol/wyntk.htm#risk

7. "National Cholesterol Education Program, Risk Assessment Toll for Estimating 10 Year Risk," accessed April 26, 2011, http://hp2010.nhlbihin.net/atpiii/ calculator.asp?usertype=prof

8. "Diabetes Pro-Professional Resources Online," American Diabetes Association, accessed May 2, 2011, http://professional.diabetes.org/GlucoseCalculator. aspx

9. "Vaccinations for Adults," CDC website on immunization schedules, last accessed May 2, 2011, http://www. immunize.org/catg.d/p4030.pdf

10. National Osteoporosis Foundation recommendations on screening, accessed May 11, 2011, www.nof. org/

11. National Cancer Institute on recommendations for screening mammograms, accessed May 11, 2011, http://www.cancer.gov/cancertopics/factsheet/detection/mammograms

www.ingramcontent.com/pod-product-compliance
Lightning Source LLC
Chambersburg PA
CBHW070231290526
45789CB00004B/1580